Prevent Stomach Ulcer

Prevent Peptic Ulcer

Read This Book And Be Informed

Olatundun Solomon

olatundunsolomon@gmail.com

Peptic ulcer is mainly caused by helicobacter pylori bacteria. This bacteria can enter the body by eating contaminated food and by drinking contaminated water. It can also enter the body by touching stool with the hands and using the hands without properly washing. When the bacteria affect the esophagus, stomach or intestine it can result to ulcer. This can cause burning sensation in the stomach and chest.

There are ways peptic ulcer can be

prevented. Examples are:

1. Prevent contaminated food.

Do not eat contaminated food. Cook food well before eating. When the food is well cooked it can prevent helicobacter pylori bacteria infection.

When food is not well cooked it can have helicobacter pylori bacteria that is living inside.

2. Prevent contaminated water.

Drink clean water. Dirty water can contain helicobacter pylori bacteria. Drinking dirty water

can cause
helicobacter pylori
infection. This can
result to peptic ulcer.
It is therefore,
important to drink
clean water.

3. Prevent touching
stool with hands and
placing into the
mouth.

Wash hands very well
with soap and water.
Also children hands
should be properly
washed with soap
and water.

4. Prevent eating
acidic food late when
you have not eaten
anything.

When food as not yet been eaten in the morning and afternoon, eating acidic food in the evening is not advisable. Acidic food can cause ulcer when it is eaten in the evening when food as not yet been eaten. Lime fruit is acidic. Cassava is acidic.

5. Prevent making the head downwards when sleeping.

Sleeping when the head is downwards can cause gastric acid from the stomach to flow to the esophagus. This can cause esophageal ulcer. This can cause chest pain. This can

cause burning
sensation in the chest.

6. Prevent eating
spicy food late when
you have not eaten
anything.

Eating spicy food in
the evening when

you have not eaten
any food can be
prevented.

7. Do exercise.

Exercise is very good
for the body. It makes
the body to be
healthy. Exercise can
make the esophagus

to be healthy.
Exercise can make
the stomach to be
healthy. Exercise can
make the intestine to
be healthy.

8. Eat vegetables.

Vegetables has
vitamins and minerals.
Eating vegetables
makes the body to be
healthy. Vitamins and

minerals increase the immunity of the body against infections.

9. Eat fruits:

Fruits as vitamins and minerals. Eating fruits makes the body to be healthy. Vitamin and minerals increase the immunity of the body against infections.

10. Sleep well.

Sleeping well makes the body to be refreshed. This makes the body to be healthy.

11. Eat whole grains.

Whole grains has fibers and nutrients. This make the body to be healthy.

12. Eat carbohydrates.

Carbohydrates gives
energy to the body.
This makes the body
to be healthy.
Carbohydrates are
wheat, barley,
potatoes and yam.

13. Eat protein.

Protein food makes growth and development to occur. Eating protein can cause repair of worn-out tissues to occur in the body. This can prevent ulcer.

14. Put vegetable oil in food.

Vegetable oil in food makes the body healthy. Vegetable oil has unsaturated fatty acid. This is very good for the body.

15. Do not smoke.

Smoking cause negative effect to the

body. It is important to stop smoking.

16. Do not drink alcohol.

Alcohol is drying agent. It is important to stop drinking alcohol.

17. Wash fruits well with clean water before eating.

When fruits are not washed, it can cause infection of the body to occur when such is eaten. It is very important to wash fruits very well with clean water before eating.

18. Wash vegetables well.

Wash vegetables well with clean water is very good. This can prevent negative effect to the body. This can prevent infection of helicobacter pylori bacteria.

19. Take your bath
with clean water.

Taking bath with dirty
water can cause
infection to the body.
It is therefore, very
important to bath
with clean water and
soap.